How I Fixed My Soft Erections Using ...

The E.D. Love Cinch

By Howard Casanova

THE E.D. LOVE CINCH IS AN EASY TECHNIQUE I USE TO...

It is my real, non-medical fix to enhance Viagra and other sexual supplements used for those embarrassing Erectile Dysfunction (E.D.) moments – one of men's biggest sexual failures!

Copyright 2015 Howard Casanova,

2nd Edition, June 2018

Casanova: The E.D. Love Cinch™

ISBN-13: 978-1796528589

ISBN-10: 1796528587

Table of Contents

What is an E. D. Love Cinch?

Simply put, it is a flexible rubber band or silicone wristband which I use to close off the blood supply to my penis (see drawing), which helps me maintain my erection.

I found the following technique worked successfully for me; for more than two years, there has **rarely been a failure...**

How I Put the E.D. Love Cinch on

IT'S **REALLY** SIMPLE TO USE!

I stretch it over either the semi- or fully- erect **penis and scrotum together** during the early or full stages of my erection – **NOT** -- when I'm still soft. The idea is to capture the entire genital area -- NOT TIGHTLY -- and, without pinching anything!

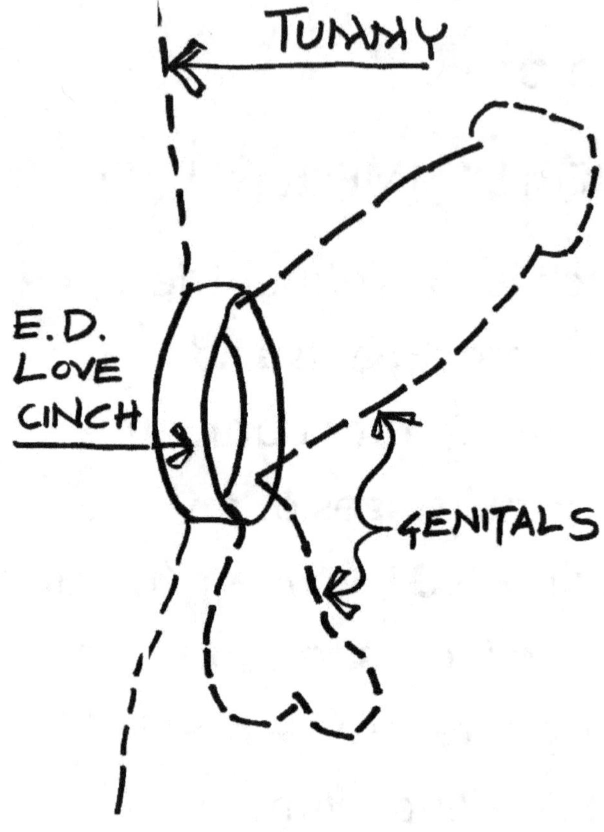

With my fingers inside the love cinch, I stretch it open... enough to slip over the **penis and scrotum** together.

Both testes must be included, as shown in diagram.

NOTE: DO NOT MISS THIS! I must be **<u>upright</u>** here (kneeling or standing) or the testis <u>cannot be captured</u>; they WILL hide in my groin.

I like to stretch it a few times to loosen it before I put it on.

It helps to be stretched first to install it correctly and (I'll repeat) -- **both testes MUST be included!**

I then adjust the love cinch for tightness and comfort without allowing it to pinch anything!

Just snug is best!

NOTE: Trimming the pubic hair around the base of my penis and scrotum makes the procedure easier. (I am VERY CAREFUL with my barber clippers here).

After much experimenting, a "wrist band," seemed to be the most logical option for the love cinch.

I Googled "wrist band" and picked out a soft silicone unit, about the size of my wrist, a little on the snug side.

Materials I have used with success include:

A vinyl/silicone wrist bracelet – (still my favorite).

Or, I also tried...

A thick *blue or red stretchy-rubber-band*, approximately 2" diameter *(like used in grocery store produce departments)*. As long as they are soft and clean.

Putting the E. D. Love Cinch to Work

With the love cinch securely in place, a few helpful tips:

BEFORE initial penetration, "**adequate** foreplay" is **strongly** suggested!

What, I had to ask is **adequate**???

WHATEVER YOUR PARTNER SAYS IT IS!

MY FIX FOR ERECTION FAILURE DURING INTERCOURSE!!!

IF, upon penetration, I feel **I am losing my erection**... **(Yikes)!** Now what?

FIRSTLY--I don't panic!

WHEN able, I simply squeeze into her and then have her close her legs together, 'underneath me', which traps my penis inside her...

I then drop both my legs to the outside of hers and slowly stroke her while she holds her legs together. This gives the penis a moment or so to fill back up. With practice, this has become a wonderful exercise for us.

Once the penis is full again (usually) in a few minutes, I'm now much ready to go, so... **WE DO!**

Benefits of the E. D. Love Cinch FOR HER!

I am NOW able to share with my partner as many orgasms as she needs to feel satisfied, *(EVEN IF I'VE ALREADY HAD MINE)* – my erection is maintained THAT much longer.

This has been the single greatest testament I can give to the love cinch.

There you have my **secrets for continual, successful sex at any age.**

My Story

I am a 70+-year young male with a severe E.D. (erectile dysfunction) condition that actually began in my 40's (*from bicycle riding, we think*). That's when my E.D. condition reared its limp, flaccid head annoyingly more often, which sadly, also left my then wife...

unfulfilled!!!

This was at about the same time that Viagra, then Cialis became popular.

I **immediately** secured a prescription from my doctor for Viagra.

It worked fantastically!

For the next 10 years or so... *until* I noticed the lessening of firmness again and a softer erection occurring more often.

Back to the doctor, who now referred me **to a urologist**. After the usual tests, it was determined (again) that I had E.D.

Now knowing of my lack of reliable success with Sildenifil Citrate (Viagra) tablets, the urologist recommended **Penile-Injections!** *(The self-injecting of Sildenifil Citrate liquid into the base of my penis with a hypodermic needle.)* **Yikes!**

However, it did work for the next year or so (painfully) ...until ALL the area around the base of my penis became uber-sensitive to ANY further injections. **Yikes (again)!**

Back to the urologist, who now recommended a "penis pump", *(like you see on late-night TV).*

This "thing" DID NOT work!

It was restrictive, painful and my orgasms were absolutely choked-off.

Back I go to the urologist who now is **quite** engaged in my problem, who refers me to radiology for an "Ultra-Sound" of my **erect** penis.

This test showed I had a **30% seepage** of blood from my erection.

Yes, this was just as weird as it sounds.

As he went over the results with me, I now understood that the blood flowed from behind my scrotum, up into the penis, (then back out the same route). Hmm...

I had an erection with a major leak!

After the failure of the penis pump and faced with this new information, I knew that **I HAD** to find a remedy! I was not about to give up on a happy, successful sex life.

I happened to be wearing a soft silicone wrist band that day and an inspiration hit me...”I wonder if that would word, I thought. I tried it, as described in this book and loved it from the first time!

And, this is how the **E. D. Love Cinch** came to be!

Happy Lovemaking!

HowardCasanova@gmail.com

NOTES

NOTES